QUICK & SIMPLE WEIGHT LOSS PLAN

By: Rolisha N. Cain

ISBN: 0615434533
ISBN-13: 978-0615434537

DEDICATION

I dedicate this book 1st to Jesus Christ, who is the author and
finisher of my faith. My loving husband
Dr. Robert Cain, and two wonderful boys
Robert Joel Cain II & Caleb Noah Cain.

CONTENTS

CONTENTS

Letter from the Author

Dear Friend,

I believe you can lose weight! Most people wish they could do something about their weight but never commit to a plan to see results. Do you really believe you can lose weight? You must believe before you achieve. Are you ready to believe in yourself and commit?

I know what it feels like to give up and not be willing to commit. I yo-yo diet for years hoping the weight will just fall off, but it didn't. The diet or weight loss plan was too complicated and I became frustrated and just quit.

I decided to research what makes people gain or lose weight. My research changed my life forever. Now I love the skin I'm in, and I'm ready to help others with the weight loss battle. If you are willing to commit, this simple plan will change your life forever!

Be Blessed & Healthy,
Rolisha Nettles Cain

Morning Inspiration

Quote this statement every morning:

Today is a new day to manage my health and weight! I will seize the day and take every opportunity to lose weight. I will walk to release my stress and think twice before I put food in my mouth, because I know a moment on my lips is a life time on my hips. No excuses! I will lose weight today!

Chapter 1 -Know Your Body

What makes your body function well? When you wake up in the morning do you feel , rejuvenated, refreshed and ready to take on the day? What do you feel like at the end of the day? Do you know how much you should weigh for your age, height, and body frame? Do you know your body?

If you don't, do not feel bad because most people don't. We live day by day hoping the weight will just drop off with no effort. We dream of being skinny like the models and actors on TV. We struggle with our mind and body daily concerning our weight and health.

Well today is the day we change our mind set. We must change our mind before our body change. When we renew our mind about our body and health we will in return lose weight.

I would like for you to write down everything you put into your body for 1 day and track the amount of sugar and carbohydrates. You will be amazed of the amount of carbohydrates and sugar you put into your body daily. Carbohydrates and sugar affects your insulin levels in your body. When your insulin levels are affected you hold fat on your hips, thighs, back of the arms and stomach. This plan will help you lose 4 to 5 pounds a week if you are willing to commit. Are you ready to know your body and lose weight?

What is Your True Size

We all have dream of being skinny and looking like someone we admire, but is their size the right size for your body. You must know your BMI. BMI is a heuristic measure of body weight based on a person's weight and height. Though it does not actually measure the amount of fat on the body, it is used to estimate a healthy body mass based on a person's height, assuming an average body composition. Due to its ease of measurement and calculation, it is the most widely used diagnostic tool to identify weight problems within a population, usually whether individuals are underweight or overweight. It was invented between 1830 and 1850 by the Belgian polymath Adolphe Quetelet during the course of developing "social physics". Body mass index is defined as the individual's body weight divided by the square of his or her height. The formulae universally used in medicine produce a unit of measure of kg/m^2. BMI can also be determined using a BMI chart.

BMI Chart

Category	BMI ranges
Severely underweight	less than 16.5
Underweight	from 16.5 to 18.4
Normal	from 18.5 to 24.9
Overweight	from 25 to 29.9
Obese Class I	from 30 to 34.9
Obese Class II	from 35 to 39.9
Obese Class III	over 40

Chapter 2- The Quick & Simple Plan

This is not a diet but a lifestyle change. You are not restricted from any food items. You can enjoy all your favorite foods, but you can ONLY have **10 grams** of sugar and **75 grams** of carbohydrates a day. Why 10 and 75, because your insulin levels will not be effected and you will lose weight. When blood sugar levels get too low, you will feel hunger. If blood sugar levels become too elevated, the pancreas secretes insulin, which lowers the blood sugar level, usually by turning it into fat. You want to maintain a constant blood sugar level to avoid feeling excessively hungry or gaining weight. Your goal with the lifestyle change is to maintain stable blood sugar levels because when sugar is released slowly into the bloodstream the body works most effectively. When blood sugar levels are kept stable, the body is able to maintain constant energy levels and you will feel fuller longer, leading to less overeating and fat loss. This lifestyle change is just that simple. Are you ready to commit?

Use the blank template on page 24 to track your grams of sugar and carbohydrates. To accelerate your weight loss, divide your 75 gram of carbohydrates by 5 and eat them throughout the day.

Example:

Breakfast: 15 gram of carbohydrates

Morning snack: 15 gram of carbohydrates

Lunch: 15 gram of carbohydrates

Mid-day snack: 15gram of carbohydrates

Dinner: 15 gram of carbohydrates

Set a Goal

Can you dream, imagine, and believe that you can lose weight? Close your eyes and imagine in your mind right now the size you desire to be. Now you must believe that you can lose weight. In order to believe you must set a goal. When there is no goal you can't track your success. When there is no success you lose your hope, which removes your faith.

What is your weight loss goal? You just can't say I want to lose weight; you must set a goal and commit to it. Most people do not set goals because they are not willing to commit. If you can't set a weight loss goal, you are not willing to commit. You will remain in your yo-yo diet mind set, always blaming others because you are not losing weight. Set a goal and write it down. Read your goal statement everyday with the morning inspiration on page 8. Your mind set will begin to change and you will lose weight.

Example of a goal statement:

I will lose 10 to 20 pound this month. I will not quit no matter what. I commit to my new lifestyle and believe all things are possible. I can and I will lose weight.

Write down your goal statement for your new lifestyle:

_____

_____

_____

_____

_____

_____

_____

_____

_____

_____

Chapter 3- Weight Loss Enemies

Stress – Friend or Enemy

Stress is a normal physical response to events that make you feel threatened or upset your balance in some way. When you sense danger – whether it's real or imagined – the body's defenses kick into high gear in a rapid, automatic process known as the "fight-or-flight" reaction, or the stress response. (Segel, 2010) We all have stress sometimes. For some people, it happens before having to speak in public. For other people, it might be before a first date. What causes stress for you may not be stressful for someone else. Sometimes stress is helpful – it can encourage you to meet a deadline or get things done. But long-term stress can increase the risk of diseases like depression, heart disease and a variety of other problems. (Health, 2010)

Do you know your stress affects your weight? When you are stressed there is a natural, stress-related hormone called cortisol that may add fat, mainly abdominal fat to your body. When you are stressed high amounts of cortisol are released into the blood stream and the receptors for cortisol are located in your abdomen, which triggers fat storage in your body. Cortisol hormones may cause your metabolism to slow down. This could mean that even if you following this plan you could gain weight because of your stress level. High stress levels also stimulates the appetite.

A daily 20 minute walk can help you release stress. Are you willing to commit to 20 minutes a day? Your mind and body will feel the differences. You could also take Saint John's Wart, which is a natural herb for stress, but please consult your doctor before taking any herbs or supplements.

Caffeine – Friend or Enemy

Research studies stated that any source of caffeine affects your adrenal gland which affects your stress levels as well. Your adrenal gland regulates your hormones while controlling your bodies' reaction to stress. When you drink coffee, which contains 100mg of caffeine per 8oz your adrenal gland automatically release hormones artificially, which produces an unnatural state of alertness. After prolonged stimulation, the adrenal glands become completely depleted and in return making your body hold fat. Do not let caffeine make you refuse to commit to your lifestyle change. Are you ready to commit?

Alternative Sweeteners- Friend or Enemy

I believe the best alternative sugar for the body is Stevia. Stevia is and herb that originated in South America. It will not cause your blood sugar level to elevate and is very sweet. I do not believe we should put chemicals in our body that are created to taste like sugar, for example: aspartame, sucarlose, and saccharin, because we do not know the long term affects it will have on our body. Most people are not affected by alternative sweeteners and alternative sweeteners should not affect your new lifestyle change on the Quick & Simple plan.

4 CHAPTER -Food Plan Examples

This chapter provides you with examples to help you with your new lifestyle change. Are you ready to wake up in the morning and feel the difference, rejuvenated, refreshed and ready to take on the day? Follow this simple plan & your body will feel the differences!

Example 1: A day on the Quick & Simple Plan

	Food Items	**Sugar**	**Carbs**
Breakfast	1 slice of toast w/ 2 eggs & 3 slices of bacon	0	9
Snack	¼ cup of blueberries	4	20
Lunch	Chef Salad	0	5
Mid-day snack	Sting cheese	0	2
Dinner	¼ cup rice Grilled chicken Veggies ½ cup of sugar free ice cream	0	25
Total		4	61

Example 2: Quick & Simple Plan (Mc Donald)

	Food Items	Sugar	Carbs
Breakfast	sausage Mc Muffin	2	29
Snack	¼ cup Nuts of your choice	0	2
Lunch	6 Piece Nuggets Garden side salad	2	20
Mid-day snack	Boston Banana Chocolate Sugar free Pudding	0	13
Dinner	Grilled Steak Broccoli & cheese ½ cup of sugar free ice cream	1	4
Total		3	68

Example 3: Quick & Simple Plan (Taco Bell)

	Food Items	Sugar	Carbs
Breakfast	2 eggs omelet Ham & cheese	0	2
Snack	Jell-O Sugar free Chocolate Mousse cup	0	10
Lunch	2 (any meat) Crunchy Tacos	2	24
Mid-day snack	Sugar free Jell-O cup	0	10
Dinner	¼ cup rice Grilled Salmon Green beans ½ cup of sugar free ice cream	0	25
Total		2	71

Example 4: Quick & Simple Plan (KFC)

	Food Items	Sugar	Carbs
Breakfast	1 slice of toast w/ 2 eggs & 3 slices of bacon	0	9
Snack	¼ cup of blueberries	4	20
Lunch	Roast Slice Turkey & cheese sandwich on whole wheat bread	0	14
Mid-day snack	¼ cup Nuts of your choice	0	4
Dinner	KFC grilled chicken Green beans & mashed potatoes w/gravy	0	21
Total		4	68

Example 5: Quick & Simple Plan (Wendy)

	Food Items	Sugar	Carbs
Breakfast	1 slice French toast w/ sugar free syrup 3 slices of bacon, 1egg	0	9
Snack	Jell-O Sugar free Chocolate Mousse cup	0	10
Lunch	Jr. Hamburger Side Salad	6	26
Mid-day snack	¼ cup Nuts of your choice	0	4
Dinner	¼ cup rice Grilled pork chops Veggies ½ cup of sugar free ice cream	0	25
Total		6	74

Blank Template:

	Food Items	Sugar	Carbs
Breakfast			
Snack			
Lunch			
Mid-day snack			
Dinner			
Total			

Your goal statement for today: *(set a goal!)*

_____

_____

_____

_____

5 CHAPTER- Low Sugar Food List

This chapter provides you with a list of items that have low grams of sugar. Remember on the Quick & Simple plan you can only have **10 grams a sugar** a day and **75 grams of carbohydrates.**

Food list items	Grams of sugar
cereals, oats, instant, fortified, plain, prepared with water	0.0
chicken roll, light meat	0.0
chicken, broilers or fryers, breast, meat and skin, cooked, fried, batter	0.0
chicken, broilers or fryers, breast, meat only, cooked, roasted	0.0

chicken, broilers or fryers, drumstick, meat only, cooked, roasted	0.0
chicken, broilers or fryers, giblets, cooked, simmered	0.0
chicken, broilers or fryers, thigh, meat only, cooked, roasted	0.0
chicken, canned, meat only, with broth	0.0
chicken, liver, all classes, cooked, simmered	0.0
chicken, stewing, meat only, cooked, stewed	0.0
coffee, brewed from grounds, prepared with tap water	0.0
coffee, brewed, espresso, restaurant-prepared	0.0
coffee, instant, regular, prepared with water	0.0
cornstarch	0.0
crustaceans, crab, alaska king, imitation, made from surimi	0.0
crustaceans, crab, blue, canned	0.0

crustaceans, crab, blue, cooked, moist heat	0.0
crustaceans, lobster, northern, cooked, moist heat	0.0
crustaceans, shrimp, mixed species, canned	0.0
duck, domesticated, meat only, cooked, roasted	0.0
fish, cod, atlantic, canned, solids and liquid	0.0
fish, flatfish (flounder and sole species), cooked, dry heat	0.0
fish, flatfish (flounder and sole species), cooked, dry heat	0.0
fish, pollock, walleye, cooked, dry heat	0.0
fish, pollock, walleye, cooked, dry heat	0.0
fish, rockfish, pacific, mixed species, cooked, dry heat	0.0
fish, roughy, orange, cooked, dry heat	0.0
fish, salmon, chinook, smoked	0.0
fish, salmon, pink, canned, solids with	0.0

bone and liquid	
fish, sardine, atlantic, canned in oil, drained solids with bone	0.0
fish, tuna, light, canned in oil, drained solids	0.0
fish, tuna, light, canned in water, drained solids	0.0
fish, tuna, white, canned in water, drained solids	0.0
frankfurter, beef and pork	0.0
frankfurter, chicken	0.0
gelatin desserts, dry mix, reduced calorie, with aspartame, prepared with water	0.0
ham, chopped, not canned	0.0
ham, sliced, extra lean	0.0
ham, sliced, regular (approximately 11% fat)	0.0
lard	0.0
leavening agents, baking powder, double-acting, sodium aluminum sulfate	0.0

leavening agents, baking powder, double-acting, straight phosphate	0.0
leavening agents, baking powder, low-sodium	0.0
leavening agents, baking soda	0.0
leavening agents, cream of tartar	0.0
leavening agents, yeast, baker's, active dry	0.0
leavening agents, yeast, baker's, active dry	0.0
leavening agents, yeast, baker's, compressed	0.0
lemonade, low calorie, with aspartame, powder, prepared with water	0.0
margarine, regular, tub, composite, 80% fat, with salt	0.0
margarine, regular, unspecified oils, with salt added	0.0
margarine, vegetable oil spread, 60% fat, stick	0.0
margarine, vegetable oil spread, 60% fat, stick	0.0

margarine, vegetable oil spread, 60% fat, tub/bottle	0.0
margarine-butter blend, 60% corn oil margarine and 40% butter	0.0
margarine-like spread, (approximately 40% fat), unspecified oils	0.0
mollusks, clam, mixed species, canned, drained solids	0.0
mollusks, clam, mixed species, raw	0.0
mollusks, oyster, eastern, wild, raw	0.0
oil, olive, salad or cooking	0.0
oil, peanut, salad or cooking	0.0
oil, sesame, salad or cooking	0.0
oil, soybean, salad or cooking, (hydrogenated)	0.0
oil, soybean, salad or cooking, (hydrogenated) and cottonseed	0.0
oil, vegetable, corn, industrial and retail, all purpose salad or cooking	0.0
oil, vegetable, sunflower, linoleic, (approx. 65%)	0.0

olives, ripe, canned (small-extra large)	0.0
pork and beef sausage, fresh, cooked	0.0
pork sausage, fresh, cooked	0.0
pork sausage, fresh, cooked	0.0
pork, cured, bacon, cooked, broiled, pan-fried or roasted	0.0
pork, cured, canadian-style bacon, grilled	0.0
pork, cured, ham, extra lean and regular, canned, roasted	0.0
pork, cured, ham, whole, separable lean and fat, roasted	0.0
pork, cured, ham, whole, separable lean only, roasted	0.0
pork, fresh, leg (ham), whole, separable lean and fat, cooked, roasted	0.0
pork, fresh, leg (ham), whole, separable lean only, cooked, roasted	0.0
pork, fresh, loin, center loin (chops), bone-in, separable lean and fat, cooked, pan-fried	0.0
pork, fresh, loin, center loin (chops), bone-in, separable lean only, cooked,	0.0

pan-fried	
pork, fresh, shoulder, arm picnic, separable lean and fat, cooked, braised	0.0
pork, fresh, shoulder, arm picnic, separable lean only, cooked, braised	0.0
pork, fresh, spareribs, separable lean and fat, cooked, braised	0.0
poultry food products, ground turkey, cooked	0.0
rice, white, long-grain, precooked or instant, enriched, prepared	0.0
salami, cooked, beef and pork	0.0
salami, dry or hard, pork, beef	0.0
salt, table	0.0
sandwich spread, pork, beef	0.0
sauce, nestle, ortega mild nacho cheese sauce, ready-to-serve	0.0
sausage, vienna, canned, chicken, beef, pork	0.0
shortening, household, soybean (hydrogenated)-cottonseed	0.0

(hydrogenated)	
snacks, pork skins, plain	0.0
soup, stock, fish, home-prepared	0.0
tea, brewed, prepared with tap water	0.0
tea, herb, chamomile, brewed	0.0
tea, herb, other than chamomile, brewed	0.0
tea, instant, sweetened with sodium saccharin, lemon-flavored, prepared	0.0
turkey patties, breaded, battered, fried	0.0
turkey roast, boneless, frozen, seasoned, light and dark meat, roasted	0.0
turkey, all classes, dark meat, cooked, roasted	0.0
turkey, all classes, giblets, cooked, simmered, some giblet fat	0.0
turkey, all classes, light meat, cooked, roasted	0.0
turkey, all classes, meat only, cooked, roasted	0.0
turkey, all classes, neck, meat only,	0.0

cooked, simmered	
veal, leg (top round), separable lean and fat, cooked, braised	0.0
vegetable oil, canola	0.0
water, municipal	0.0
soup, vegetarian vegetable, canned, prepared with equal volume water, commercial	1.4
oat bran, raw	1.4
broccoli, frozen, chopped, cooked, boiled, drained, without salt	1.4
potatoes, mashed, home-prepared, whole milk and margarine added	1.4
cauliflower, cooked, boiled, drained, without salt	1.4
potatoes, baked, skin, without salt	1.4
broccoli, cooked, boiled, drained, without salt	1.4
cucumber, peeled, raw	1.4
lima beans, immature seeds, frozen, baby, cooked, boiled, drained, without	1.4

salt	
lime juice, canned or bottled, unsweetened	1.4
lime juice, canned or bottled, unsweetened	1.4
lima beans, immature seeds, frozen, fordhook, cooked, boiled, drained, without salt	1.3
kale, frozen, cooked, boiled, drained, without salt	1.3
cheese, swiss	1.3
asparagus, cooked, boiled, drained	1.3
bread, pita, white, enriched	1.3
bread, pita, white, enriched	1.3
sauce, ready-to-serve, pepper or hot	1.3
kale, cooked, boiled, drained, without salt	1.3
cheese, pasteurized process, swiss, with di sodium phosphate	1.2
beans, snap, green, frozen, cooked, boiled, drained without salt	1.2

beans, snap, yellow, frozen, cooked, boiled, drained, without salt	1.2
lettuce, cos or romaine, raw	1.2
soup, bean with pork, canned, prepared with equal volume water, commercial	1.2
potato, baked, flesh and skin, without salt	1.2
snacks, corn-based, extruded, chips, plain	1.2
cheese, muenster	1.1
egg, whole, cooked, hard-boiled	1.1
worthington foods, morningstar farms burger "crumbles "	1.1
alcoholic beverage, wine, dessert, dry	1.1
asparagus, canned, drained solids	1.1
cauliflower, frozen, cooked, boiled, drained, without salt	1.1
cheese, mozzarella, whole milk	1.0
pumpkin, cooked, boiled, drained, without salt	1.0
cheese, parmesan, grated	1.0

crackers, rye, wafers, plain	1.0
garlic, raw	1.0
artichokes, (globe or french), cooked, boiled, drained, without salt	1.0
artichokes, (globe or french), cooked, boiled, drained, without salt	1.0
snacks, tortilla chips, plain, white corn	1.0
beans, snap, green, canned, regular pack, drained solids	1.0
beans, snap, yellow, canned, regular pack, drained solids	1.0
beef stew, canned entree	1.0
alcoholic beverage, wine, table, white	1.0
soup, onion, dehydrated, prepared with water	1.0
crackers, melba toast, plain	1.0
lettuce, butterhead (includes boston and bibb types), raw	0.9
cereals ready-to-eat, wheat, shredded, plain, sugar and salt free	0.9

lettuce, butterhead (includes boston and bibb types), raw	0.9
baking chocolate, unsweetened, squares	0.9
parsley, raw	0.9
buckwheat groats, roasted, cooked	0.9
snacks, rice cakes, brown rice, plain	0.9
tortillas, ready-to-bake or -fry, corn	0.9
fast foods, chicken, breaded and fried, boneless pieces, plain	0.9
snacks, popcorn, air-popped	0.9
potatoes, boiled, cooked in skin, flesh, without salt	0.9
potatoes, boiled, cooked without skin, flesh, without salt	0.9
potatoes, boiled, cooked without skin, flesh, without salt	0.9
bread, italian	0.9
cabbage, chinese (pak-choi), cooked, boiled, drained, without salt	0.8
egg, whole, cooked, fried	0.8

barley, pearled, raw	0.8
lettuce, green leaf, raw	0.8
spaghetti, whole-wheat, cooked	0.8
egg, whole, cooked, poached	0.8
egg, whole, raw, fresh	0.8
egg, whole, raw, fresh	0.8
gravy, nestle, chef-mate country sausage gravy, ready-to-serve	0.8
gravy, chicken, canned	0.8
egg, whole, raw, fresh	0.8
turnip greens, frozen, cooked, boiled, drained, without salt	0.8
wild rice, cooked	0.7
egg, white, raw, fresh	0.7
snacks, popcorn, cakes	0.7
tofu, soft, prepared with calcium sulfate and magnesium chloride (nigari)	0.7
fast foods, potato, french fried in vegetable oil	0.7

soup, chicken noodle, canned, chunky, ready-to-serve	0.7
cornmeal, whole-grain, yellow	0.6
cornmeal, degermed, enriched, yellow	0.6
egg substitute, liquid	0.6
alcoholic beverage, wine, table, red	0.6
soup, beef noodle, canned, prepared with equal volume water, commercial	0.6
tofu, firm, prepared with calcium sulfate and magnesium chloride (nigari)	0.6
seaweed, kelp, raw	0.6
cheese, mozzarella, part skim milk, low moisture	0.6
soup, cream of mushroom, canned, prepared with equal volume water, commercial	0.6
beet greens, cooked, boiled, drained, without salt	0.6
bread, pumpernickel, toasted	0.6
collards, frozen, chopped, cooked, boiled, drained, without salt	0.6

soup, vegetable beef, prepared with equal volume water, commercial	0.6
worthington foods, morningstar farms better'n burgers, frozen	0.6
cheese, provolone	0.6
macaroni, cooked, enriched	0.6
spaghetti, cooked, enriched, without added salt	0.6
snacks, popcorn, oil-popped, microwaved	0.5
egg, yolk, raw, fresh	0.5
bread, pumpernickel	0.5
cheese, cheddar	0.5
cheese, low fat, cheddar or colby	0.5
cheese, feta	4.1
mushrooms, shiitake, cooked, without salt	4.1
carrots, frozen, cooked, boiled, drained, without salt	4.1
corn, sweet, white, cooked, boiled,	4.1

drained, without salt	
spices, oregano, dried	4.0
peas, edible-podded, boiled, drained, without salt	4.0
nuts, pecans	4.0
carambola, (starfruit), raw	4.0
carambola, (starfruit), raw	4.0
pasta with meatballs in tomato sauce, canned entree	4.0
tomatillos, raw	3.9
sauce, barbecue sauce	3.9
cereals ready-to-eat, general mills, cheerios	3.9
cabbage, red, raw	3.9
carrot juice, canned	3.9
bread, rye	3.8
healthy choice beef macaroni, frozen entree	3.8
snacks,tortilla chips, nacho-flavor	3.8

soup, cream of mushroom, canned, prepared with equal volume milk, commercial	3.8
soup, tomato, canned, prepared with equal volume water, commercial	3.7
nuts, pine nuts, dried	3.6
chicken pot pie, frozen entree	3.6
nuts, pine nuts, dried	3.6
salad dressing, blue or roquefort cheese dressing, commercial, regular	3.6
corn, sweet, yellow, frozen, kernels on cob, cooked, boiled, drained, without salt	3.6
cabbage, raw	3.6
pizza, cheese topping, regular crust, frozen, cooked	3.6
corn, sweet, yellow, canned, vacuum pack, regular pack	3.6
tomato juice, canned, with salt added	3.6
english muffins, plain, enriched, with ca prop (includes sourdough)	3.5
pickles, cucumber, dill	3.5

cocoa mix, with aspartame, powder, prepared instant	3.5
english muffins, plain, toasted, enriched, with calcium propionate (includes sourdough)	3.5
carrots, cooked, boiled, drained, without salt	3.4
frankfurter, beef	3.4
peppers, sweet, green, cooked, boiled, drained, without salt	3.4
tapioca, pearl, dry	3.3
squash, winter, all varieties, cooked, baked, without salt	3.3
cowpeas, common (blackeyes, crowder, southern), mature seeds, cooked, boiled, without salt	3.3
pumpkin, canned, without salt	3.3
vegetable juice cocktail, canned	3.3
soup, pea, green, canned, prepared with equal volume water, commercial	3.3
corn, sweet, yellow, canned, cream style, regular pack	3.2

cowpeas (blackeyes), immature seeds, cooked, boiled, drained, without salt	3.2
seaweed, spirulina, dried	3.2
eggplant, cooked, boiled, drained, without salt	3.2
corn, sweet, yellow, cooked, boiled, drained, without salt	3.2
vegetables, mixed, frozen, cooked, boiled, drained, without salt	3.2
crackers, standard snack-type, sandwich, with cheese filling	3.1
bread, reduced-calorie, wheat	3.1
corn, sweet, yellow, frozen, kernels cut off cob, boiled, drained, without salt	3.1
sauce, ready-to-serve, salsa	3.1
soup, clam chowder, new england, canned, prepared with equal volume milk, commercial	3.0
soybeans, mature cooked, boiled, without salt	3.0
spices, curry powder	3.0

snacks, oriental mix, rice-based	3.0
turnips, cooked, boiled, drained, without salt	3.0
cabbage, cooked, boiled, drained, without salt	2.9
kellogg's eggo lowfat homestyle waffles	2.9
lima beans, large, mature seeds, cooked, boiled, without salt	2.9
peas, split, mature seeds, cooked, boiled, without salt	2.9
okra, frozen, cooked, boiled, drained, without salt	2.9
mung beans, mature seeds, sprouted, cooked, boiled, drained, without salt	2.8
pimento, canned	2.8
kohlrabi, cooked, boiled, drained, without salt	2.8
mustard, prepared, yellow	2.8
snacks, pretzels, hard, plain, salted	2.8
snacks, corn-based, extruded, puffs or twists, cheese-flavor	2.8

dandelion greens, cooked, boiled, drained, without salt	2.7
cheese, cottage, lowfat, 1% milkfat	2.7
seeds, sunflower seed kernels, dry roasted, with salt added	2.7
seeds, sunflower seed kernels, dry roasted, with salt added	2.7
tomatoes, red, ripe, raw, year round average	2.7
tomatoes, red, ripe, raw, year round average	2.6
tomatoes, red, ripe, raw, year round average	2.6

References

Dietary Fiber. (2009). *Low Sugar*. Retrieved December 1, 2010, from Dietary Fiber Food: http://www.dietaryfiberfood.com/

Eknoyan, Garabed (January 2008). "Adolphe Quetelet (1796-1874)—the average man and indices of obesity". *Nephrol. Dial. Transplant*. 23 (1): 47–51. doi:10.1093/ndt/gfm517. PMID 17890752.

E.g., the Body Mass Index Table from the NIH's NHLBI. Health, N. I. (2010, September). *Stress*. Retrieved November 12, 2010, from Medline Plus: http://www.nlm.nih.gov/medlineplus/stress.html

Segel, J. (2010, November). *Understanding Stress- Signs, Symptoms, Causes, and Effects*. Retrieved December 28, 2010, from Help Guide http://helpguide.org/mental/stress_signs.htm

Disclaimer

The Information in this book is for educational purposes only. It is in no way intended to replace the knowledge or diagnosis of your professional health care/nutrition attendant.